VERY LITTLE

IS NEEDAD

TO MAKE

A HAPPY LIFE,

IT IS ALL WITHIN

YOURSE LF, IN

YOUR WAY OF

THINKING

.........................MARCUS AURELIUS.........................

www.ingramcontent.com/pod-product-compliance
Lightning Source LLC
Chambersburg PA
CBHW070126290526
45789CB00005B/2145
* 9 7 8 1 5 3 7 4 1 0 0 4 3 *